The word YOGA means 'union'
meditation during your pregnan
equilibrium and unity of mind and body.

In each of us there is a deep centre where primordial and instinctiveknowledge comes from. Yoga will bring you into direct experience ofthis inner centre and help you to get in touch with your power andpotential for giving birth and mothering.

There are also many physiological benefits to the muscular, skeletal, respiratory, circulatory, excretory and nervous systems of the body.When you practice yoga regularly you will soon notice an improvementin your health and vitality. By enhancing your own health you are also providing the best possible nourishment for your baby at this vital stageof his or her development.

Yoga encourages emotional release and is a great aid to quietening and calming restless or anxious states of mind. It can be invaluable in helping you to cope with any difficulties that may arise before during and after birth and to make the most of the joyous and blissful times and the natural tendency to turn inwards during your pregnancy.

As you learn to flow with the rhythm of your breathing your body will gradually come into harmony with gravity. This will improve your posture and help you to feel more centred, while increasing your trust in your body's ability to surrender to the involuntary processes that will bring your baby to birth.

It will also deepen your awareness of the inner connection you have with your child and enhance your communication during the months before and after birth.

To download the MP3 of Yoga instructions
narrated by Janet go to:
www.activebirthcentre.com/downloads
and use the download code: YFP16

HOW TO USE THE MP3

PREPARING

Start by downloading the MP3 from the link on page 1 and prepare to play it. Choose a time of day when you are unlikely to be disturbed. The complete session takes about 2 hours and can be done in one go if you have the time. Or you can use it for several separate sessions of a series of postures each throughout the week, or in any way that you find convenient.

You will need to work in a warm well-ventilated room on a carpeted floor, or else use a non-slip yoga mat and a folded blanket for the kneeling positions. Some of the positions are done against a wall, so try to make a free wall available in the room you are using for your practice. It is best to practice in the same place every day with the few things you need close at hand. You may need a soft belt; a blanket; two small cushions; one large cushion and a low stool or pile of large books. Plants, flowers, candles or an agreeable incense or essential oil can help to enhance the experience.

Make sure you eat something light an hour or two before practising, but never do yoga immediately after a heavy meal. Follow your practice with a drink of herbal tea or fruit juice before resuming your usual activities.

Bathing in warm water or swimming before doing yoga will help to loosen your body and increase flexibility, especially first thing in the morning when muscles and joints tend to be a little stiff.

WHAT THE MP3 INCLUDES

The MP3 consists of a complete session of yoga practice. Part One begins with deep breathing and this is followed by a sequence of basic yoga postures and movements which are suitable for any stage of pregnancy. The postures are clearly illustrated by the drawings on the following pages and described by the instructions on the MP3. You will find that each exercise begins with details of how to place your body and is followed by suggestions for breathing while in the posture. The same deep breathing, as in the first exercise, is used throughout to help you to relax and release tension. The sessions end on Part Two with some meditation and relaxation.

CAUTIONS

It is important to read the cautionary notes in the booklet carefully before beginning each posture. If you have any chronic pain, such as back pain or any bleeding or other complication in your pregnancy it is essential to consult your doctor before starting this programme, to ensure that these exercises are recommended. Generally, the exercises are perfectly safe for all women to practice during pregnancy and will improve health, regulate blood pressure and help to ease most ailments or minor discomforts. However, every body is different. Always listen to what your body tells you and stop if a particular movement feels unpleasant or painful.

Some women find that they are uncomfortable lying on their backs during pregnancy, particularly in the last 8 weeks. This is because the weight of the heavy uterus presses on the large blood vessels in the abdomen, which may slow down circulation and cause dizziness. If this is the case, come out of the posture slowly and, in future, leave out all the exercises which involve lying on the back.

Similarly, some women find that standing positions or forward bends should not be held for too long while others enjoy staying in them for a few minutes. At all times let your body be your guide. Stop to rest whenever you have had enough and leave out any movement which is unsuitable.

Sometimes releasing muscular tension can also bring up memories or strong feelings and emotions. These may relate to the present or may have been held inside or suppressed for a long time. If this happens, then stop listening for a while to allow the feelings to surface and continue when you feel ready.

STARTING

Relax while the introductory music is playing, becoming calm and quiet before you begin. Start on Part One with "Deep Breathing". Try to follow the instructions the first time around but, expect to take several sessions before your breathing deepens and becomes effortless. Continue with the postures in sequence, as they unfold on the MP3, concentrating on becoming familiar with the positions. To avoid confusion, you may prefer not to follow the breathing instructions at first. Start by familiarising yourself with the postures and simply breathe in the normal way. When the postures are familiar, the breathing instructions will begin to make sense. This will probably take a little time, but with regular practice the MP3 will become easy to follow and use throughout your pregnancy.

In some cases, for example, "Deep Breathing" or "Pelvic Floor Exercises" there is a choice of alternative positions illustrated in the booklet. Simply choose the one you find most comfortable and easiest for your body, using the pause button to try them out at your leisure when you start. It is natural to feel a little tightness, tension or stiffness when you first begin to use these postures. Some are bound to be more comfortable than others, but the more testing ones are probably the ones you need the most and they will become easier with practice.

It is important to avoid straining and to allow your body time to gently relax into each of the positions. Pace yourself according to your own limits and leave out any posture that causes undue discomfort.

TIMING

The timings on the MP3 for each track are designed to be comfortable for daily practice. In the beginning, especially if this is the first time you are doing yoga, you may wish to stop before the time allowed. If this is the case, then listen to your body and stop when you feel like it - gradually increasing the time you spend in each position. On the other hand, after working with the MP3 for some time, you may wish to extend the pauses between positions and stay longer in each one. This can easily be done by using the pause button.

TAKING IT EASY

Once you get to know them, all the yoga postures and exercises on this MP3 should be easy to do. If this is the first time you are experiencing this type of exercise, allow yourself a few weeks to understand how it works. The drawings in this booklet illustrate the full posture but don't expect yourself to be able to do all of them completely in the beginning. It will take time for your body to loosen up sufficiently. Simply go as far as you can comfortably manage without straining and then relax and breathe. It doesn't matter if your knees or hands don't touch the floor yet, or that some movements are less easy than others - the important thing is to follow the instructions carefully and gently within your own limits. Your awareness of the positions and breathing will grow at its own pace. Always follow your own natural rhythm using the instructions as a general guide.

Yoga is a passive and non-strenuous form of exercise. It involves becoming comfortable in certain postures, going only as far as your own natural limits will take you. As soon as you feel any strain you are going too far. Each position brings you into balance and harmony with the earth's gravitational force by focusing your awareness on the way your body contacts the floor and using your breathing to deepen this awareness. As you breathe you will become aware, at first, of your own inner centre and then of the relationship of your body to the ground. As you become more connected both to your inner sense of self and the earth, you will feel more 'grounded', calmer and more secure, and your general posture and health should improve.

At first you are bound to encounter the stiffness that has accumulated in your body. Gradually you will become aware of an increasing sense of relaxation and ease in the postures. Your joints and muscles will become more flexible, aided by the help of gravity and the hormones you secrete in pregnancy, to make your body more supple for birth. You will be learning to release unnecessary tension and tightness as you breathe. During your pregnancy this will help you to recover your original suppleness and to go beyond your usual limits. It is also the best way to prepare for releasing tension during strong contractions in labour and to stay fit and healthy before and after the birth.

Try to bear in mind, as you practice, that yoga is all about surrendering to the natural relaxed state that is already there, in all of us, behind the accumulated tension and resistance. In the same way that it took a long time to build up the tightness, it is going to take time to gradually release it. It is not about trying to achieve the perfect posture. Once you have understood the principle of slowly letting go, rather than trying, your practice is well under way!

Part I

TRACK 1

DEEP BREATHING

Choose your sitting position finding the one which is most comfortable (a, b, c, or d). Place a folded blanket or small cushion underneath your buttocks or sit with your lower back supported by a wall. If your knees do not touch the floor place a small cushion under each knee.

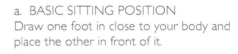

a. BASIC SITTING POSITION
Draw one foot in close to your body and place the other in front of it.

b. SITTING WITH LEGS OUTSTRETCHED
Place your legs comfortably apart and relax.

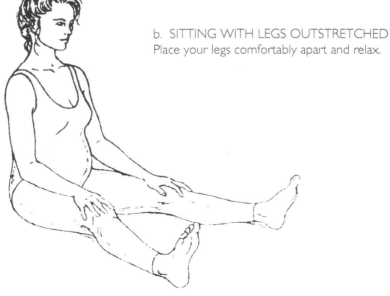

c. HALF LOTUS

Draw one foot in close to your body. Place the other one on top of it with the sole of the foot turned up and the toes resting on the opposite thigh.

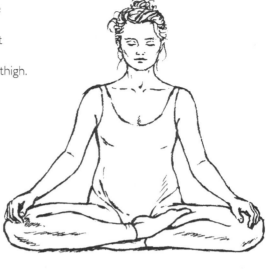

d. LOTUS

Use this position only if you have very supple knees, hips and ankles. Bend both knees and then, one at a time, place each foot on the opposite thigh in the crease of the groin with the sole facing up.

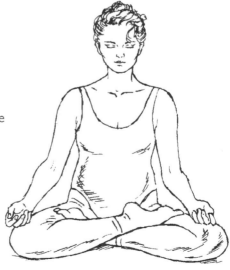

TRACK 2.

LEG STRETCH
Draw one foot in close to your
body and extend the other leg.
Use a soft belt to catch your foot.

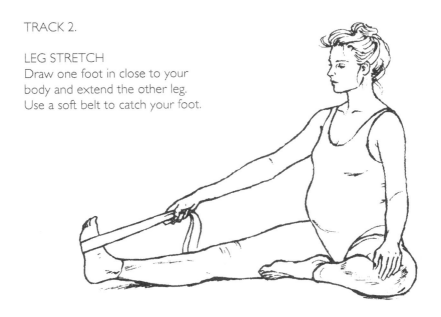

TAILOR POSE
Bend your knees and bring
the soles of your feet together.
Sit with your back supported by
a wall if you prefer.

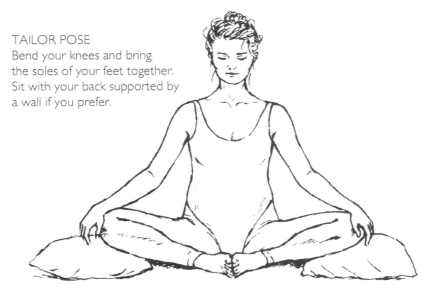

SITTING WITH LEGS WIDE APART
With legs as wide as possible, relax your thighs and extend your heels. Sit with your back supported by a wall if you prefer.

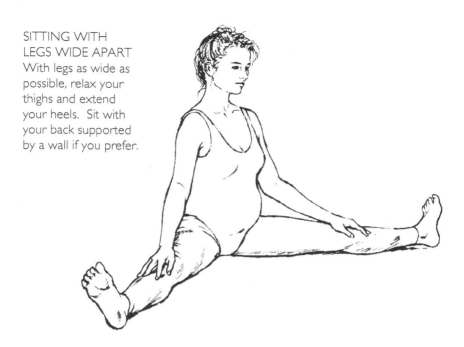

COMING FORWARD
Caution: Only do this movement when your hips are loose enough to bend forward keeping your back straight, hips down and your spine free.

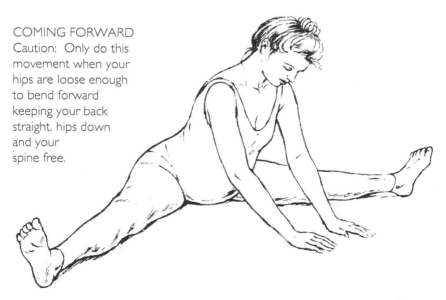

TRACK 3

PELVIC RELEASE
a. Sitting on the heels.
With your knees apart, turn your
feet inwards with your toes facing
towards the centre.

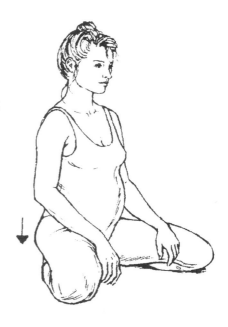

b. Level I
Keep your pelvis on your
heels and come forward
onto your hands.

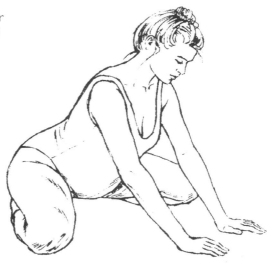

c. Level 2

With a straight back, come forward
onto your elbows. Place a large
cushion underneath your trunk
for level 2 and 3 if it is more
comfortable.

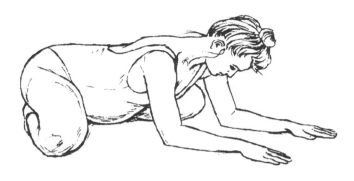

d. Level 3

Keep your pelvis down and stretch
out and place your forehead on the floor

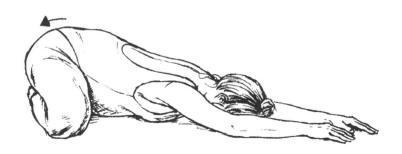

TRACK 4

BASIC KNEELING
POSITION
With knees together
sit on or between your
feet. Turn your toes in
towards the centre.

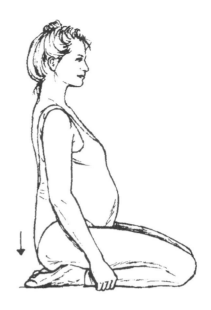

SPINAL TWIST
Lengthen your lower
back and tuck under
your pelvis

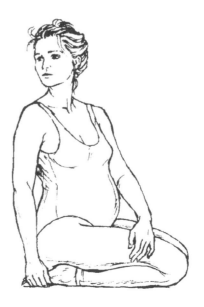

PELVIC LIFT
Lengthen your lower
back and lift your pelvis.

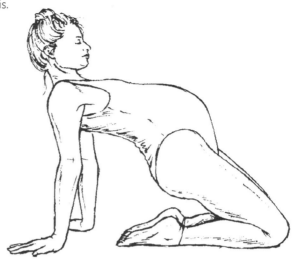

ALL FOURS TUCK-IN
Lengthen your lower
back and tuck under
your pelvis.

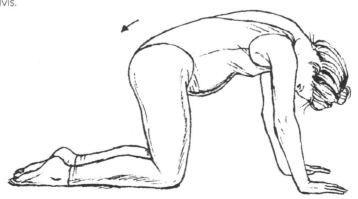

TRACK 5

MOVEMENTS FOR LABOUR

a. HANDS AND KNEES
Roll your hips in slow
sensuous circles.

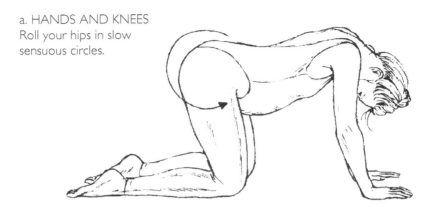

b. UPRIGHT KNEELING
Come onto your knees
and roll your hips.

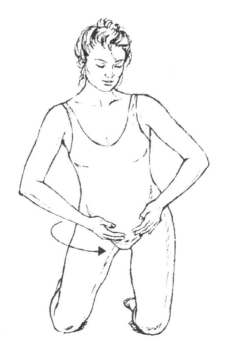

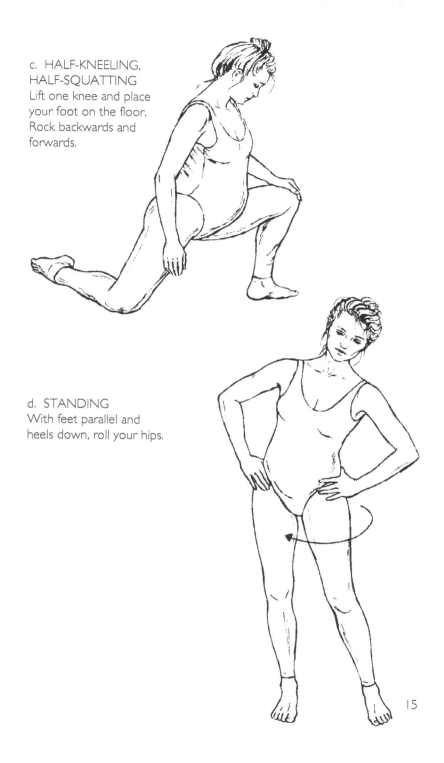

c. HALF-KNEELING,
HALF-SQUATTING
Lift one knee and place
your foot on the floor.
Rock backwards and
forwards.

d. STANDING
With feet parallel and
heels down, roll your hips.

15

TRACK 6

BASIC STANDING POSITION
When standing or walking always place your feet parallel by turning
your heels out and your toes in slightly with the outside edges of your
feet in line. Lengthen your lower back so that your pelvis tucks under.
Relax your neck and shoulders. Drop your weight into your heels.

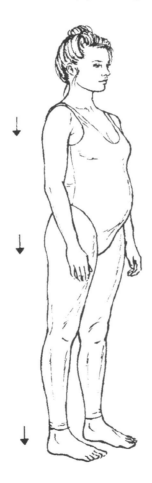

a. BACK NECK STRETCH
Bring your head forward.
Clasp your hands behind
your head and gently bring
your elbows down.

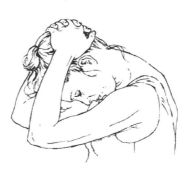

b. FRONT NECK STRETCH
Let your head hang back and
bring your teeth together.

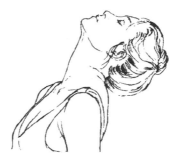

HEAD ROLL
Roll your head around
making slow circular
movements.

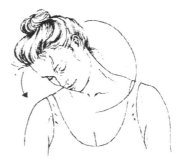

TRACK 7

FORWARD BEND

CAUTION: Due to circulation
changes, a few women
experience discomfort or
dizziness when bending
forward or in the standing
postures. If this is the case:
- use position (ii) instead of (i)
- or stay in the posture only briefly
- or leave the exercise out altogether.
Avoid bending forward if you have
haemorrhoids or piles.

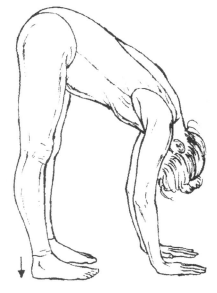

a. FORWARD BEND Position (i)
With your heels down, bend forward
from the hips. Bend your knees to
come up

b. FORWARD BEND Position (ii)
Use a table for support so that your arms and upper body are
horizontal and your neck relaxed.

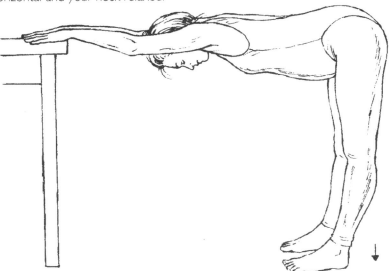

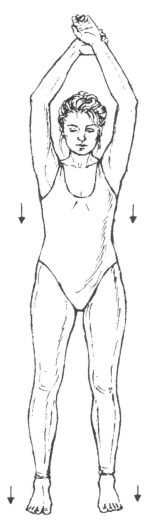

TRACK 1

SHOULDER RELEASE
WITH ARMS UP
Lift your arms keeping your lower back
long, your heels down and your
shoulders relaxed.

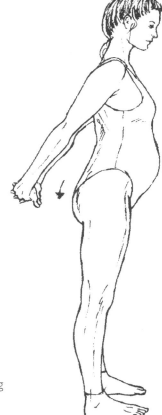

b. SHOULDER RELEASE
WITH ARMS BACK
Link your fingers behind your back and bring
your arms up so that your shoulder blades
come towards the centre of your back.

19

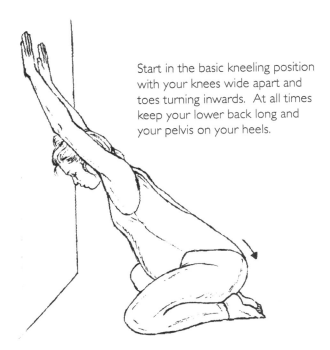

Start in the basic kneeling position with your knees wide apart and toes turning inwards. At all times keep your lower back long and your pelvis on your heels.

c. SHOULDER RELEASE ON THE WALL

d. CHEST RELEASE WITH PALMS TOUCHING
In the basic kneeling or standing position, place your palms together up the centre of your back..

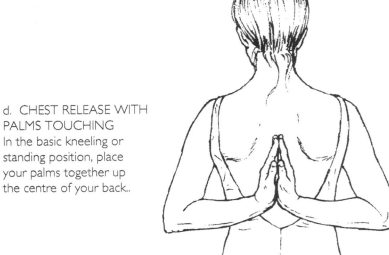

e. CLASPING THE HANDS
Clasp your fingers with the top elbow pointing up to the ceiling and the bottom elbow to the floor.

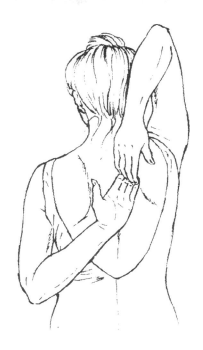

f. HAND CLASP USING A BELT
Use a soft belt if your hands do not touch.

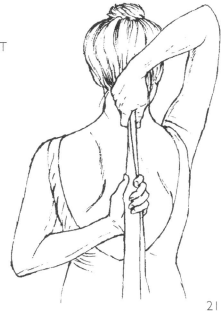

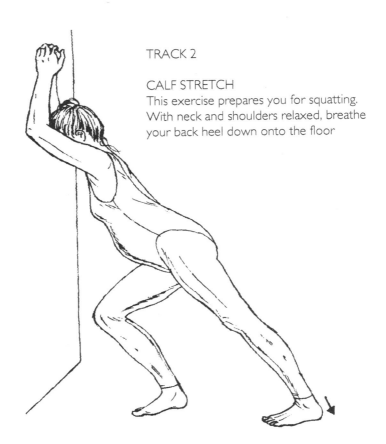

TRACK 2

CALF STRETCH
This exercise prepares you for squatting.
With neck and shoulders relaxed, breathe
your back heel down onto the floor

SQUATTING
Choose the most comfortable
position for squatting from a, b
and c.
Caution: Avoid full squatting if
you have varicosities or a cervical
stitch and use position c.
If your baby is in the breech position
after 34 weeks, avoid squatting
altogether.

a. FULL SQUAT
With heels flat on the floor
and knees apart, lift the arches
of your feet.

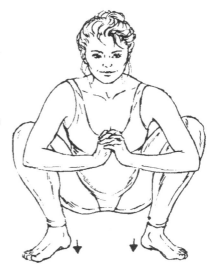

b. SUPPORTED SQUAT

If a. is difficult, use b. for a
few weeks and then try again.
Use a firm support to
keep your heels down and
elbows straight with the
knees wide apart.

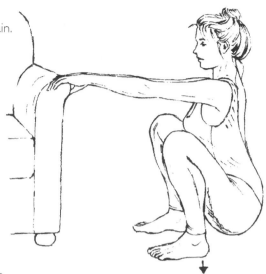

Suggestion: Place a rolled up
yoga mat under your heels.

c. SQUATTING ON A STOOL

Choose this position if you
have haemorrhoids (piles)
or a cervical stitch.

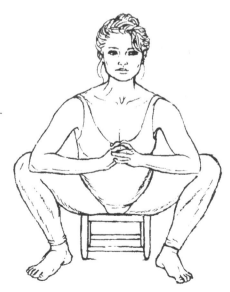

PELVIC FLOOR EXERCISES

Choose the most suitable position
from a, b, c, and d. Your pelvic floor
muscles lie like a hammock across
the base of your pelvis. The fibres
run in a double figure of eight pattern
to surround your urethra,
vagina and anus. Your baby
will come down the birth
canal and pass through
these muscles when he
or she is born. It is
important to keep
them in good tone.

a. EASY SQUATTING
Squat on your toes using
your hands for support.
Change to b, or d as needed

b. KNEE-CHEST POSITION
Caution: Choose this position
if you have vulval or anal
varicosities or if your baby
is in the breech position
after 34 weeks.

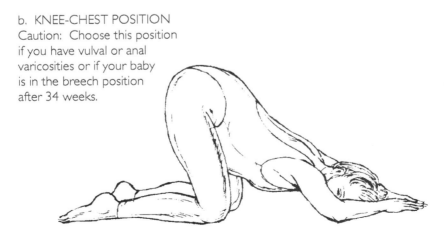

c. HALF-KNEELING, HALF-SQUATTING
Kneel and then lift one leg and place the foot on the floor.

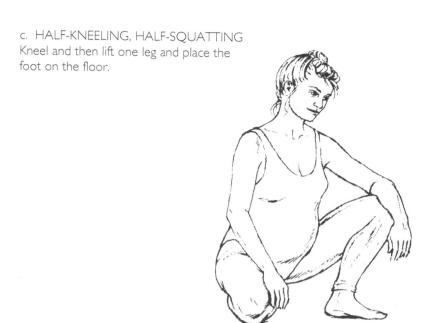

d. ALL-FOURS.
Kneel on your hands and knees.

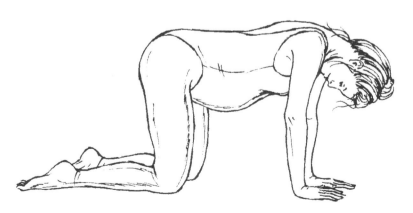

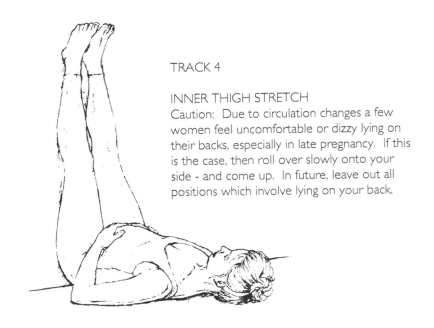

TRACK 4

INNER THIGH STRETCH
Caution: Due to circulation changes a few women feel uncomfortable or dizzy lying on their backs, especially in late pregnancy. If this is the case, then roll over slowly onto your side - and come up. In future, leave out all positions which involve lying on your back.

a. STARTING POSITION
Start by sitting down sideways next to the wall and then lie down. Your buttocks should touch the wall. Relax and release your spine.

b. LEGS WIDE APART
Let your legs open out to the side as wide as possible.

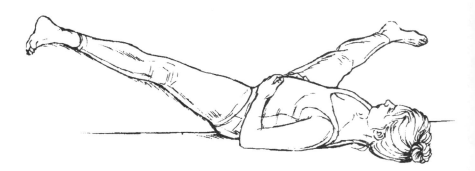

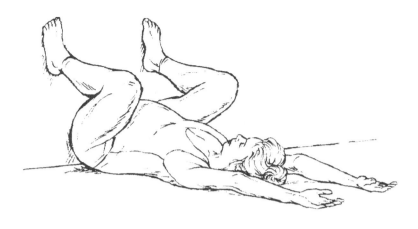

c. RESTING POSITION
Bend your knees, as if squatting, to rest.

d. TAILOR POSE ON THE WALL
Bring the soles of your feet together. Use your hands to gently press your knees towards the wall.

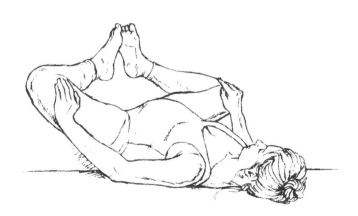

SPINAL TWIST

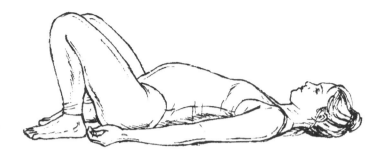

b. Look towards one hand and then turn your knees gently in the opposite direction.

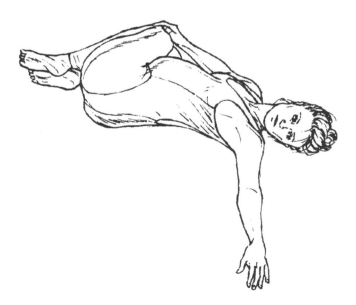

TRACK 6

RELAXATION AND BABY MEDITATION
Lie on your side. Make sure you are completely comfortable placing a
cushion under your head and another between your knees. If it is cold,
cover yourself with a warm blanket before you start.

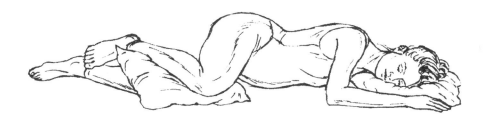

Yoga and Narration
Janet Balaskas

Drawings
by Lucy Su

Design
by
Fiona Douglas

Music: Part One
Bach Concerto in D Minor for Violin and Oboe
Movement II 'Adagio'
Menuhin/Goosens

Part Two
'Dawn Chorus' from 'The Big Field'
Music for acoustic guitar, dobro and mandolin
by Piérs Partridge

Digital Recording by Jay Burnett

ACKNOWLEDGMENTS
I would like to thank yoga teachers
Mina Semyon and Sandra Sabatini
for their inspiration.

Thanks to Jocelyn James
for allowing us to photograph and sketch
her yoga practise.

My gratitude to Yehudi Menuhin
and Piers Partridge
for the music
and
Jane and Jay Burnett for the recording

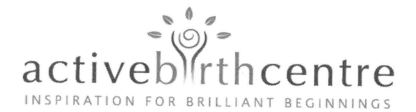

activebirthcentre

INSPIRATION FOR BRILLIANT BEGINNINGS

Janet teaches at the Active Birth Centre in London. Her approach is inspired by the teachings of Vanda Scaravelli, which bring awareness of gravity, the breath and the gentle unfolding and lengthening of the body to yoga practice.

This is a way of doing yoga that liberates both body and mind and helps us to find balance, inner peace and connection with ourselves and others.

It is especially suitable and safe for pregnancy, and is wonderful preparation for birth and motherhood.

To find a register of trained Pregnancy Yoga and
Active Birth Workshop Teachers go to

www.activebirthcentre.com

Active Birth Centre
25 Bickerton Road
London N19 5JT
Tel: 0207 281 6760
Info@activebirthcentre.com

Discover a wealth of beneficial
information, inspiration and resources...
Learn how you can make informed choices,
and gain the confidence to be actively in charge of
your pregnancy, birth and early parenting.

Made in the USA
San Bernardino, CA
03 May 2016